HEALTH

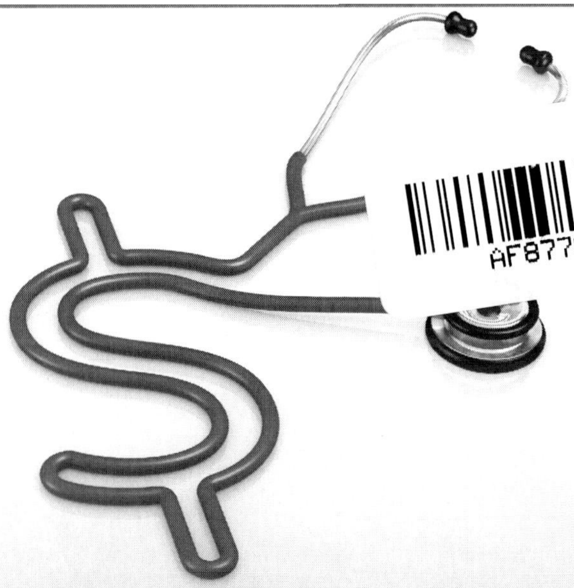

How America Sold Out On Health Care

Second Edition

René Ryman

HEALTH CARELESS:
HOW AMERICA SOLD OUT ON HEALTH CARE
by René S. Ryman

The views and opinions expressed within this book are not necessarily that of those persons, institutions, organizations, or places that have been mentioned or interviewed.

Published by

OUT of the BOX

Out of the Boxx, Inc.
OutOfTheBoxx.com

Cover and interior by Nick Zelinger, NZGraphics.com

ISBN: 978-0-9743504-2-4 (print)

LCCN: 2019920269

Second Edition

Printed in the United States of America

Contents

"The American Republic will endure until politicians realize they can bribe the people with their own money."

— Alexis de Tocqueville

From the Author

Have you ever experienced or witnessed unfair claims processing from an insurance company? Perhaps you or someone you know has suffered financial hardship because of an injury or illness. Yet while insurance industry profits soar, the number of uninsured in the United States has been steadily rising each year. Even in cases of clear liability for payment of medical expenses and damages, insurance companies are dodging their responsibilities by using strong arm tactics, political posturing, and expensive legal teams – all at the expense of rising premiums for the dwindling number of policyholders. While insurance industry profits have risen significantly, well over a million Americans have been forced into bankruptcy due to unpaid medical expenses.

I have published several articles about the insurance industry, including one entitled "*The Top Ten Reasons Why It Is Great To Be An Insurance Company*" that ran in newspapers across the country in the fall of 2003. For months I was besieged and overwhelmed with responses to that article. I heard from people from all walks of life who were insured yet were unable to get medication for their terminally sick children, retired people on fixed incomes who never planned on a 600 percent increase in their insurance payments, and most commonly those from Middle America who had to choose between feeding their families or purchasing insurance coverage and prescriptions. I can honestly say that I never expected this kind of response to an article that I wrote simply to vent my own frustrations with the current health care system.

I do not consider my experiences unique or more deserving than any other case. However, as a writer and researcher I felt compelled to take a closer look at our health care system, which is designed to build shareholder profit at the expense of patient care. Many politicians (mostly Republicans) believe that government should not get into the business of health care any more than it already is. Is this in the best interests of the citizens of the United States, or in the best interests of the insurance industry that makes significant campaign contributions to elected state and federal officials? I am perplexed by the fact that the U.S. government can run a large military operation entrusted with nuclear devices that could wipe out an entire nation, but somehow feels that the responsibility of running a health care system is beyond its capability.

This book will evaluate many of the factors that are challenging the patients, the uninsured, and those who are on the brink of financial hardship because of health care expenses. This book will also reveal those other less than flattering contributors to the demise of affordable and adequate coverage for Americans.

Top Ten Reasons Why It's Great to Be an Insurance Company

1. *You can still make money during a recession.*
Travelers Property Casualty Corporation's net profit jumped 33 percent in the second quarter of 2003. Travelers' Chairman and CEO, Robert I. Lipp, responded about the earnings that "outstanding results this quarter demonstrate the earnings power of the company."[1]

2. *You can still increase premiums while many don't have insurance.*
Today 41.2 million Americans have no health insurance. A Kaiser Family Foundation survey showed that the average annual insurance premium for a family of four increased 13 percent to $7,954 in 2002, up from $7,053 in 2001; annual coverage for individuals increased by 15 percent, from $2,650 in 2001 to $3,060 in 2002.[2]

3. *You can bully state regulators to give you what you want.*
PacifiCare of Colorado threatened to withdraw from the market if lawmakers did not pass insurance-industry regulatory reforms. Principal Life Insurance Co. and other insurance providers considered taking a similar stance.[3]

In Rhode Island, John Alden Life Insurance Company joined the list of companies exiting the state, citing burdensome regulation. Conseco, Inc. said it would close down its last major medical insurance unit and end coverage for about 40,000 members in 20 states.[4]

4. ***You don't care if hospitals close because you can make money without them.***
The number of private hospitals in the U.S. decreased 7 percent over a 20-year period, from 4,052 in 1980 to 3,759 in 1999. During that time, the number of public hospitals dropped 33 percent, from 1,778 to 1,197.[5]

5. ***You don't have to worry about paying claims on time.***
A poll conducted by the Harvard School of Public Health revealed that nearly half of the respondents had problems with their health plan that included delays and denials of care and receipt of payment for services rendered.[6]

6. ***Your adjusters can use unethical tactics to not pay claims.***
Insurers often fail to adequately investigate claims, they deny claims without supporting evidence, they make unreasonably low settlement offers, they refuse to reveal policy limits, they refuse to negotiate, they make oppressive demands not required by the policy, they destroy evidence that would support the insured's claim for benefits, and they rely on minor misrepresentation in the insurance application to deny coverage or to coerce acceptance of a claim.[7]

7. ***Your adjusters can deny claims and more than 50 percent of claimants won't challenge it.***
In May 2003, HomeCare, Inc. mailed reimbursement

questionnaires to 1,500 randomly selected domestic subscribers. The results revealed that 6 to 10 percent of the claims submitted were denied by the insurance provider and 44 percent of these denied claims were appealed.8 Nationally, 40 percent to 60 percent of insurance providers' decisions are overturned.[9]

8. ***If you are accused of low-balling claims, you can blame it on the computer.***

More than 40 property and casualty insurers use the Colossus system as a knowledge-based tool for adjusters in evaluating personal injury claims.[10] Farmer's parent company, Zurich Financial Services Group, revealed that in one year of operation, Colossus had reduced claims about 20 percent.[11]

9. ***Your investors and the public will never know about your bad faith activity.***

Punitive damages for bad faith claims against insurance companies are one million dollars in more than one-third of the verdicts. The mean punitive damages award is $4.9 million. This is in addition to compensatory damages, which in bad faith cases are awarded for "emotional distress."[12] These amounts for bad faith lawsuits and settlements are passed on to policyholders through premium charges. Currently, regulators do not require insurance companies to break down their expenses in their financial reports to disclose to shareholders and policyholders the amounts paid for settlements and verdicts.[13]

10. ***Your future looks even brighter!***
Robert I. Lipp, Chairman and CEO of Travelers Property Casualty Corporation, promised investors that he was determined to make his company "better than most" in the property/casualty sector.[14]

1

A Brief Review of the American Health Care System

The health care spending in the United States rose to $1.6 trillion in 2002 and grew 5.7 percent faster than the overall economy as measured by Gross Domestic Product (GDP).[15]
— Centers for Medicare & Medicaid Services

History reveals that insurance coverage dates back to ancient Egyptian times as it was known to have existed around 3000 BC when Chinese merchants dispersed their shipments among several vessels to avoid the possibility of severe damage or the total loss of their cargo.[16] Further evidence shows establishment of an insurance system referred to as the "Code of Hammurabi," which was derived from the practices of Babylonian traders and was used by early Mediterranean sailing merchants. The Greeks and Romans lived in societies where coverage for funeral expenses was provided by benevolent citizens as a matter of cultural practice. Insurance evolved when a variety of coverage policies became available to those seeking protection during the post-Renaissance Europe.[17]

There are some insurance companies in existence in the United States today that were actually started in the mid 1700's and who provided relief to banks during the 1930's and the Great Depression.[18] Benjamin Franklin, an American printer, author, philosopher and scientist, helped to popularize and set standards of practice for insurance coverage. In the nineteenth century the U.S. government sought to deregulate the industry to allow a variety of financial institutions, including banks, the opportunity to sell insurance policies.[19]

Initially physicians engaged in a direct business relationship with their patients. Doctors provided care based on a fee schedule that was designed to offer services that were affordable to those seeking care. This system allowed doctors to control their conditions of practice and fees, and enabled patients to freely select the doctors of their own choice.[20] This allowed physicians to control their incomes, and patients to select and continue health care treatment with their preferred providers.

While the United States continued with private insurance, prior to the start of World War I most European countries had established nationalized health care programs as a way to manage insurance costs and, in addition, to regulate the level of care provided to patients. The focus of these national health care programs was (and is) to consider:

1) individual loss of income,
2) individual medical costs,
3) indirect costs of illness to society, and
4) social costs of medical care.[21]

Overall, the success of a national program is to focus on a variety of issues within the health care system that contribute to quality and accessible medical treatment.

During the 1920's and 1930's a few organizations began offering "medical operatives" as a way to offer medical care to groups of participants. Organizations such as the Los Angeles Department of Water and Power implemented an employee plan that offered treatment for their employees at the Ross-Loos Clinic, a full service medical clinic owned by Dr. Donald Ross and Dr. H. Clifford Loos. Yet, even as more employees and groups sought to join the growing number of medical cooperatives, the American Medical Association (AMA) became uneasy about this new form of patient care that was unregulated. AMA administrators threatened to seek reprisals against any doctors who participated in these plans and sought to punish them by preventing them from obtaining admitting privileges at certain hospitals.

In 1938, the AMA was indicted on charges for violating the Sherman Act, and the following year 26 states formally passed legislation that prevented consumer-run medical services plans. Under the new law, medical service plans had to be formed by doctors who would then oversee the programs, and all new plans had to be approved by the state medical society where services were provided.[22]

Medical insurance plans offered by employers gained popularity during World War II when employers offered health care coverage to attract potential employees. The number of Americans who enrolled in health coverage programs grew from seven million prior to the start of the war, to more than 26 million as new jobs were created during the war.[23] Because companies were prohibited from granting wage increases and were under strict price controls during the war, health care coverage was offered as a fringe benefit to employees, and by 1955 enrollment piqued at 101 million participants.[24]

At the same time (between the years of 1934 and 1954), labor union membership experienced its most substantial growth, and political power of the unions was firmly established nationwide. It was during this era that membership grew from 3 million to 18 million. During this period (from 1947 to 1954), real wages for unionized production workers increased an average of 3.0 percent a year. After World War II ended and the need to offer hiring incentives diminished for employers, labor unions began to include health care in the negotiations for collective bargaining strategies.[25]

In 1965 Medicare and Medicaid were signed into law with the purpose of providing health care services to the poor and elderly who did not have access to other medical insurance plans. In the late 1960's and early 1970's politicians and interest groups began promoting proposals to reform the nation's health care system.[26] Paul Ellwood, M.D., who is considered the 'modern day father of the HMO concept,' created and promoted 'health maintenance organizations' (or HMO's as they are more commonly known to the general public) that offered an option of managed care plans. Dr. Ellwood convinced President Nixon's aides to formulate a health care policy whereby a "nationwide system of prepaid group practices and foundations for health care would link a system capable of being most cost efficient and thus provide an answer to the country's health care problems."[27]

The Health Maintenance Act of 1973 was passed into law, and after several amendments to the legislation over the next few years, Dr. Ellwood's policy for improved quality through competition in for-profit HMO plans grew its participants from 12 percent in 1981 to approximately 62 percent in 1998.[28] HMO's, along with 'preferred provider organizations' (PPO's), both offer to participants managed care through pre-selected doctors and medical treatment facilities. Today critics of the system believe the well-intended model for better health care has become a primary revenue source for business interests and corporate profits.[29]

The United States health care system is today one of the fastest growing contributors to the Gross National Product (GNP). Between 1998 and 2002, health care costs spiked 35 percent, and critics claim that there is no evidence to show any changes that will slow the growth of health care spending.[30]

Today the United States has approximately 45 million uninsured,[31] and rising insurance premiums will more than likely continue to eliminate those who are able to afford health care coverage.[32]

Since the first printing of this book in 2005, the most significant change to the U.S. health care industry was the enactment of the Affordable Care Act (ACA) on March 23, 2010. The program was launched October 1, 2013 as an alternative to private health care companies with the goal of providing health care for all Americans. However, as the cost of health continues to rise – the following updated data reflects a continual increase in expenditures through 2016.

	1980	1990	2000	2016
National Health Expenditures (billions)	$245.8	$696.0	$1,310.0	$3,328.0
Health Expenditures as a Percentage	8.8	12.0	13.3	17.9
Health Expenditures per capital	$1,067	$2,738	$4,178	$10,348

2016 data retrieved from https://www.healthaffairs.org/doi/abs/10.1377/hlthaff.2017.1299 July 25, 2018.

2

French Revolution Health Care Crisis – Yes, It's Happened Before!

"Access to hospital care should be equally available to all Frenchmen irrespective of where they live." [33]
— *The French Revolution and the Poor*, Alan Forest

The health care crisis the United States is now experiencing is similar to the one that occurred more than two centuries ago in France and that directly contributed to the start of the French Revolution in the late 1700's. The call for freedom and equality were central Revolutionary tenets. They found full expression when feudalism was abolished with the decree of August 26, 1789 that clarified the Rights of Man and the Citizen and resonated concerns about pre-revolutionary agendas for medical change.[34]

Before the Revolution, provision of health care to French citizens was unequal and depended greatly on wealth and social status. The quality of care was somewhat equal for everyone because truly great advancements in medicine had not yet begun. In the sixteenth century, for example, during the outbreak of the plague, the medical treatment for disease was equal across income levels due to the lack of medical advancements and medicines. Similarly, all other things being equal, the plague was as prone to kill a prince as a pauper.[35] Nevertheless, a member of the royal family had greater access to the most learned doctors than did ordinary citizens.

At that time, many hospitals in France were Catholic charitable foundations that had evolved from humble medieval beginnings.[36] Hospitals were places of refuge for the lower classes of society and were shunned by people of even modest means.[37] Doctors probably treated far more paupers in hospitals than they did in private practice. Although doctors did take on charity cases, the vast bulk of their clients were from the middle and upper classes who could afford their fees.[38]

To obtain health care in those days, one needed to be either poor enough to be eligible for charity or wealthy enough to afford to pay for services with out-of-pocket funds. Many working-class citizens could not afford to pay for health care.[39] A sliding scale was available based on personal income, but the costs were still beyond the means of most workers. In some regions, physicians' fees were fixed by statute, but even then only patients who were fairly well off could afford the fees for medical treatment, which often equaled the daily wage of an agriculture worker or modest artisan.[40] Cash was scarce, and many practitioners were often obliged to accept payment in kind. Often they were not paid at all, and more than likely, fees for those who could afford to pay were increased to cover such bad debts. Many preventable illnesses and deaths occurred because affordable health care was lacking.[41]

Although the Revolutionary call for equality was noble, the effect of the French Revolution itself on the nation's already feeble health care system was disastrous. Charitable giving to hospitals dried up after the Revolution broke with the Catholic Church in 1790. Potential donors were only further discouraged when Revolutionary administrators insisted on re-allocating funds received from benefactors away from health care expenses and instead used the money for their own purposes.[42]

To make matters even worse, wounded and ill soldiers from the war front descended on civilian hospitals in search of medical attention. Payment for expenses incurred from caring for military personnel invariably arrived months late and failed to cover the quickly rising treatment costs.[43] Panic among health care providers arose. Hospitals could not afford to both feed patients and pay for routine supplies – they could not afford to stay in business.[44]

The need for reform was apparent. Without some kind of intervention, France stood to lose health and medical care altogether for virtually all of its citizens. Because the French government recognized the threat and took action, the number of hospitals that ultimately were actually forced to close was very small.[45]

The French Revolution is prominently mentioned in the history of medicine. A transition to socialized medicine began in France after the French Revolution and was based on Revolutionary principles.[46] In the years that followed the French Revolution, during the reign of Emperor Napoleon Bonaparte, the word of the day was "equality," and equality in health care was no exception. Napoleon embraced a series of goals to revolutionize the state's role in tending to citizens' health.[47] The birth of socialized medicine in France became part of the new social reform. Napoleon insisted that access to hospital care should be equally available to all Frenchmen, regardless of where they lived. The money to pay for the care would come out of the central tax structure.

Beginning in 1791, several million livres were voted every year for hospital management; it was paid to health care departments on the basis of their population levels for reallocation to the various hospitals in their territory.[48]

Overall, this new system constituted a nationwide and rationally ordered system of health care delivery. The cost structure was made uniform, and patients were permitted to choose their health care providers. The liberal values of the revolutionaries were fundamentally endorsed: the rights of physicians to practice freely, and of patients to freely choose their doctors, were uncontested.[49]

Repeating History in the United States

The United States is currently experiencing a health care crisis not unlike that of pre-revolutionary France. In the United States today, low-cost or no-cost care is available to the indigent and the elderly, and the well-to-do can afford all the health care that money can buy. But a large (and growing) percentage of ordinary wage earners cannot afford health insurance, and without health insurance, they cannot afford even basic levels of care. In 2001, 43 million Americans had no health insurance.[50] Thus, in terms of access to medical treatment, the gap between the haves and the have-nots is widening.

Unlike in pre-revolutionary France, most states in this country require emergency rooms to admit all comers. Those who cannot otherwise afford health care quickly learn this. The cost of providing emergency medical services to emergency room patients who ultimately do not pay their bills is passed on to those who can. "People without insurance go to doctors and emergency rooms anyway," says Larry Boress, executive director of the Chicago Business Group on Health, a purchasing coalition of 70 local companies. "When they don't pay their bills, the cost of their care is shifted indirectly to big companies and their insurers, who do pay the bills. The uninsured have played a role in raising costs of health insurance for everybody else who is covered." Higher health care costs result in higher health insurance premiums.[51]

Even workers accustomed to employer-paid health insurance are feeling the pinch. Hewitt & Associates, a global human resources outsourcing and consulting firm, reported that in 2002 many companies passed on at least 25 to 30 percent of their premium increases to employees, which means increases ranging from $186 to $463 per month. The report found that employers are expecting average annual premium increases over the next few years of about 13 percent, but they are only willing to pay 8 percent of that increase. "You look at that kind of gap and ask who is going to pay for it, and the answer is the employee," said Ken Sperling, Hewitt's health care practice leader.[52]

Nationally, a Kaiser Family Foundation survey showed that the average annual insurance premium for a family of four increased 13 percent to $7,954 in 2002, up from $7,053 in 2001. The cost of coverage for individuals increased by 15 percent, from $2,650 in 2001 to $3,060 in 2002.[53]

Contrary to public perception, the medically uninsured and underserved aren't clustered in homeless shelters or soup kitchens. Many work long and hard hours, but either their paychecks do not allow for deductibles or co-payments, or their employers have been priced out of the health insurance market.[54] "Eight out of 10 uninsured Americans are in working families," said John J. Sweeney, president of the AFL-CIO. "They can't afford health insurance on their own if their employers do not provide it or if they are asked to shoulder a big share of the premium."[55]

The percentage of working-class individuals who are uninsured is growing, and younger people make up an increasing part of the group of uninsured. The state of Georgia has estimated that 1.3 million of its residents – about 8 percent of the state's population younger than 65 – do not have insurance. "An average increase of 8 percent in annual premiums for Georgia's private businesses, which is double the present inflation rate, could bring the number of uninsured to more than 1.5 million by 2005," according to Ken Thorpe, an Emory University health policy expert.[56]

In Illinois in 1999, according to U.S. Census Bureau estimates, 14 percent of residents did not have health insurance. Of the uninsured, 65 percent were between the ages of 19 and 39, and only 35 percent were 40 to 64 years old.[57]

Like France during its Revolution, the United States is struggling to keep hospitals open as health care costs spiral out of control. The number of private hospitals in the United States decreased 7 percent over 20 years, from 4,052 in 1980 to 3,759 in 1999. Also during that period, the number of public hospitals dropped a whopping 33 percent – from 1,778 to 1,197.[58]

In this country, state insurance regulators are charged with the responsibility of protecting the public from catastrophic disasters in our health care system. As a practical matter, however, insurance regulators and state legislators do the bidding of the hugely powerful insurance industry. While premium costs continue to rise, while the number and percentage of uninsured citizens increases, and while hospitals struggle to stay open, the insurance industry gets state regulators to approve higher and higher health insurance premiums by threatening to eliminate all medical coverage unless rate increases are approved.

In 2001, for example, Colorado's largest health insurer, PacifiCare of Colorado, threatened to withdraw from the small-group health insurance market if Colorado lawmakers did not pass insurance industry regulatory reforms. Principal Life Insurance Company made a similar move, and other insurance providers considered taking comparable stances in states that did not pass favorable reforms. An estimated 480,000 Coloradoans are included in the small-group insurance market, and PacifiCare insures 50,000 of those.

"Unless there is meaningful legislative change this year, we will approach the Division of Insurance to discuss steps that might offer some relief," said Val Dean, president and chief executive officer of PacifiCare of Colorado.[59]

The insurers' threats are not idle. When state regulators refuse to budge, insurers actually do pack and leave. In Rhode Island, for example, health insurer John Alden Life Insurance Company – a subsidiary of Milwaukee-based Fortis Health – joined the list of companies exiting the state, citing burdensome regulations. "It's a culmination of events that started a year ago with extensive regulatory mandates and regulations being overlaid. It became impossible for us to stay," according to spokesman Robert Guilbert.[60] He declined to say which specific regulations he was referring to.

In 2002, Conseco, Inc. said it would close down its last major medical insurance unit and end coverage for about 40,000 members in 20 states. According to spokesman Mark Lubbers, "Eventually you may see three or four carriers serving each market."[61] If further regulation is unacceptable to the remaining insurance providers, we can expect them to exit the insurance business as well, leaving many more citizens without coverage.

According to Democratic Senator John Breaux of Louisiana, "We have to fundamentally change the health care system in this country. The current system is in chaos and it's getting worse."[62] Today more and more Americans must choose: no health care coverage, or reduced coverage at higher out-of-pocket rates. The United States has some of the finest doctors and medical facilities available, but a growing number of Americans do not have access to this expertise. Immediate action is needed to correct this trend.

Recently, the United States has experienced a trend toward a socially funded medical system. In addition to the federally funded Medicare/ Medicaid programs, HHS Secretary Tommy G. Thompson has provided grants to 20 states to develop plans to provide their uninsured with affordable health insurance.[63] "It is vital that we work to expand access to health insurance to all our citizens," said Secretary Thompson.[64]

The State of Tennessee has addressed the issue of its health care crisis by the implementation of a state-run managed care program providing coverage to more than 1.4 million residents, including those who are uninsured and uninsurable. The New Hampshire Department of Health Services currently provides health care to more than 80,000 residents and is seeking to expand coverage to more of its residents.[65]

In conclusion, the state of the U.S. health care system is that taxpayers have been funding socialized health care without realizing it and without many receiving its benefits. Government expenditures accounted for about 60 percent of total U.S. health care costs in 1999, according to a Harvard Medical School study published in the journal *Health Affairs*.[66] According to Steffie Woolhandler, a study author and an associate professor of medicine at Harvard, "We pay the world's highest health care taxes. Every other developed nation has national health insurance. We already pay for it, but we don't get it."[67]

In 2005, approximately 45 million Americans did not have health insurance. Since the enactment the Affordable Care Act (ACA) on March 23, 2010, there has been a significant reduction of uninsured Americans since the plans roll out in 2013. The following will review the annual change in the number of uninsured relative to the age categories (up to age 65) of those who have health insurance coverage.

US PUBLIC HEALTH CARE COVERAGE UNDER AGE 65 2013-2016

Year	Pop USA	Uninsured	Under age 65 with public coverage	Age 18-64 with public coverage	Under age 18 with public coverage
2013	313,401	41MIL	23.80%	16.70%	42.20%
2014	316,168	33 MIL	24.50%	17.70%	42.20%
2015	318868	29 MIL	25.30%	18.90%	42.20%
2016	320372	27.3 MIL	26.30%	20.00%	43.00%

* Public coverage info: *https://www.cdc.gov/nchs/nhis/releases.* htm retrieved July 15, 2018
**Demo info: *https://www2.census.gov/programs-surveys/demo/ tables/p60/260/table6.pdf*
retrieved July 15, 2018

3

Insurance Company Bad Faith: The Real Culprit Responsible for Rising Insurance Premiums

Insurance companies regularly blame across-the-board premium increases on a combination of inflation and jury verdicts that they claim are out of control. Premium increases due to increases in the costs of underlying goods and services (e.g., medical care, car repairs) are legitimate and unavoidable, but insurance company dollars spent campaigning for so-called "tort reforms" to avoid high jury verdicts would be better spent on reforming their own claims handling practices. Mandatory reporting of the claims payments and the components thereof would go a long way toward solving the mystery with respect to how much inflation is to blame and how much insurance companies themselves are to blame.

Insurance Premium Increases Are Outpacing Inflation

Insurance premiums continue to increase faster than the rate of inflation while coverage steadily decreases, pricing many unfortunate consumers, especially those on low or fixed incomes, out of the market. The insurance industry would have us believe that the rate increase is merely keeping pace with the rising cost of medical care and automobile parts. In fact, the rate increases have outpaced by a wide margin increases in the cost of the goods, and will continue to do so in the future.

For example, health insurance premiums rose 11 percent between 2000 and 2001, according to the Kaiser Family Foundation and Health Research and Education Trust.[68] The California Public Employee's Retirement System – the nation's largest health insurance plan after the federal government – announced a premium increase of 25 percent. However, the change in the Consumer Price Index – All Urban Consumers, U.S. City Average, Medical Care, from 2000 to 2001 – was only 4.6 percent.[69]

"Tort Reform" Is Not the Answer

When confronted with the reality that insurance premium increases are outpacing inflation in the cost of the covered goods and services, insurance companies usually blame the civil justice system, claiming that jury verdicts are too high. They call for "reforms" in the civil justice system, at least insofar as remedies for torts that they insure are concerned.

Colorado was one of the first states to be hoodwinked. Insurers spent millions of dollars on advertising to convince the public that the near doubling of insurance premiums in the mid 1980's was due to high personal injury damage awards. Many suspect that the real reason for the "crisis" was insurance companies' lower returns on investments due to lower interest rates. The advertising and lobbying campaign succeeded. In 1989, the Colorado legislature enacted laws:

- Abolishing joint and several liability (parties that are responsible and/or at fault) in favor of "pro rata liability."
- Reducing statutes of limitations, reducing – and in some cases, eliminating – workers' rights under workers' compensation statutes.
- Granting immunity for governmental agencies and for some special interest groups, capping damages for non-economic damages in personal injury cases to $250,000 (or $500,000 if there is a clear and convincing justification), adjusted annually for inflation in some, but not all, cases.
- Limiting medical malpractice awards to $1 million, for which no more than $250,000 may be awarded for non-economic damages, without adjustment for inflation, but with the proviso that the $1 million limit may be exceeded based only upon a showing of good cause, and
- Limiting punitive damages to an amount not in access of actual damages, with the ability to reduce that amount if the wrongful conduct has ceased, or to increase it to no more than three times actual damages if the wrongful conduct has not ceased.

A few years later the Colorado legislature eliminated the ability to obtain punitive damages in wrongful death cases and limited non-economic damages in wrongful death cases to $366,250. Personal injury cases in Colorado dropped from 5,793 in 1986 to 3,444 in 1987. But by 1991 they increased again to 6,054, more lawsuits than were filed before the law changed.[70] After three years of living under tort reform, Colorado citizens began to understand how they have been duped. The legislation did not result in lowered premiums, increased availability of insurance coverage, or simplification of the system. It did, however, return profitability to the insurance industry in spades.[71]

Today Coloradoans continue to face significant rate increases and the backlash of tort reform if they are involved in a lawsuit. "Rate increases are averaging 15 percent to 20 percent," said Carole Walker, executive director of the Rocky Mountain Insurance Information Association, a non-profit insurance group.[72] "We have gone too far," said Sen. Al Meiklejohn, R-Arvada. "Some of it needed to be done, but we shouldn't hurt Colorado citizens in the process."[73]

In 1989, at the request of Rep. James J. Florio, D-NJ, chairman of the House Subcommittee on Commerce, Consumer Protection and Competitiveness, the U.S. General Accounting Office examined the profitability of the automobile insurance industry over a 10-year period. The agency's report, issued in October '89, said that after-tax profits of the industry were about $22.6 billion dollars in 10 years. The property and casualty industry had $374 billion in assets in 1986 with a net worth of $94 billion and profits of $12.1 billion. Not bad for an industry in "crisis."[74]

Poor Claims Handling Is to Blame

In an effort to attract policyholders, insurance companies use marketing campaigns to give policyholders the impression that "they'll be there for you," observed Bob Horkovich, a partner with Anderson Kill Olick & Oshinsky in New York.[75] Allstate promises, "You're in good hands." Still, Allstate felt the need a few years ago to commence a public advertising campaign designed to convince policyholders that they do not need to hire a lawyer to represent their interests. State Farm promises that "Like a good neighbor, State Farm is there," but State Farm is no stranger to bad faith claims. Recently, State Farm appealed a $145 million punitive damages jury verdict against it to the U.S. Supreme Court. In that case, the jury found State Farm liable for bad faith, fraud, and intentional infliction of emotional distress.[76]

A "bad faith" claim exists when an insurance company fails to honor its obligation to its policyholder. Policyholders assume that when they submit a claim their insurers will negotiate in good faith and compensate them fairly for their losses. Yet in too many cases, claims adjustors deny legitimate claims or use strong arm tactics to entice claimants to take less than they are entitled to receive under their insurance policies. According to Bob Horkovich, "Insurers are gambling that you might back out and they might win."[77]

Claimants know that they can either settle for less than that to which they are entitled or face a lengthy legal process to recover the actual amount of damages owed to them. According to Horkovich, "Insurers also realize that because

98 percent of bad faith suits never go to trial, they can collect interest on money paid in premiums."[78] This further entices adjusters to dig in their heels when paying claims. "They hold on to it, earning interest. That's bad faith," stated Horkovich.[79]

Too often, insurers fail to adequately investigate claims, deny claims without adequate supporting evidence, make unreasonably low settlement offers, refuse to reveal policy limits, refuse to negotiate, make oppressive demands not required by the policy, destroy evidence that would support the insured's claim for benefits, reject the recommendations of counsel regarding settlements, and rely on minor misrepresentations in the insurance application as a reason for denying coverage, or to coerce acceptance of a compromise of a claim.[80] They have many ways to stonewall a claim.

When the breach of the promises made in the insurance policy is particularly egregious, and a great many have been, juries are permitted (subject to the so-called "tort reform" laws) to award punitive damages. The policy behind punitive damages, of course, is to make it hurt so that the insurance company will not do it again.[81]

The money and effort spent by the insurance companies securing "tort reform" would be better spent on reforming their own claims handling practices. According to the Jury Verdict Research Series, the average mean of punitive damages for bad faith claims is $1 million. The report further states that 53 percent of the claims result in awards for more than $1 million. Jury Verdict Research Series identifies about 500 bad faith cases against insurers that went to verdict between 1986 and 1992. Punitive damages were awarded in more than one-third of the verdicts. This is on top of compensatory damages, which in bad faith cases are awarded for "emotional distress."[82]

A review of insurance bad faith verdicts in California from 1991 to 1999 reveals that punitive damages constitute 77 percent of all the damages imposed by juries against insurance companies for breach of the covenant of good faith and fair dealings. Punitive damages were awarded in 42 percent of the cases, which is substantially higher than the 4 to 6 percent rate of punitive damages in all civil litigation. In those cases in which punitive damages were awarded, the mean punitive damage award was $16,655,895 and the median punitive damages award was $2,816,000.[83] The amount of these verdicts for substantial punitive damages, coupled with attorney fees, expert witness fees, and other associated court costs, is passed on to the policyholders.

Better Reporting and Oversight Is Needed

Insurance companies are clearly not regulating themselves adequately when it comes to honest claims paying practices. Better state regulation is in order. State regulators should shine a bright light on claim payment practices by requiring insurers to provide better and more detailed reporting of bad faith claims. This should hopefully cause claims adjusters to think twice before denying legitimate claims. Fewer bad faith claims should result in smaller rate increases.

At the present time, insurance companies do not break down their claims expense in their financial reports to their shareholders and policyholders. There is no way of knowing what percentage of "claims and claims expenses" or "other costs and expenses" consists of punitive damage awards and defense costs as compared to covered goods and services. In this era of questionable accounting practices, it would be appropriate for regulators and shareholders to insist on a more detailed accountability to ensure ethical management practices. Insurers should be required to report bad faith lawsuits and their outcomes (whether by settlements or verdict) to state insurance regulators.

Insurers should also be required to itemize their claims expenses in their financial reports with greater detail. For example, legal fees for defending insureds should be segregated from legal fees for defending the insurance company itself. Sums paid to insureds or third parties for covered claims should be stated separately from sums paid to insureds in settlements or satisfaction of bad faith claims.

This chapter reviewed tort reform as many states have aggressively revised statutes in favor of capping recovery of damages in injury cases. However, the Obama administration did not support such reforms and maintained that awards and recovery of damages should be left to the judicial process on a case by case basis without such limitations.

Since President Trump became President of the United States, a new trend has emerged with House Republicans introducing bills that would make changes to the civil justice system long sought by doctors and U.S. corporations, including a cap on some medical malpractice awards and implementing new roadblocks designed to deter claims for seeking compensation for medical injuries and associated losses.

According the data in this chapter regarding political contributions and lobbying efforts we note that between 2002 (page 42) and 2015 there was a significant increase in the amount of an increase of $71.5 million. The lobbying efforts increased between 2000 (page 42) to 2016 in the amount of $46.5 million. In 2016, the highest year for political contributions dollars, it was also the year of the largest annual increase of insurance premiums.

> "Capping malpractice payments . . . would do nothing to prevent unsafe practices or ensure the provision of fair compensation to patients . . .
>
> Apology offered by a health care provider during negotiations shall be kept confidential and could not be used in any subsequent legal proceedings."
>
> — Hillary Clinton & Barack Obama[1]

This chapter reviewed tort reform as many states have aggressively revised statutes in favor of capping recovery of damages in injury cases. However, the Obama administration did not support such reforms and maintained that awards and recovery of damages should be left to the judicial process on a case by case basis without such limitations.

Since President Trump became President of the United States, a new trend has emerged with House Republicans introducing bills that would make changes to the civil justice system long sought by doctors and U.S. corporations, including a cap on some medical malpractice awards and implementing new roadblocks designed to deter claims for seeking compensation for medical injuries and associated losses.[2]

[1] Hillary Rodham Clinton & Barack Obama,(2006) *Making Patient Safety the Centerpiece*, 354 N. ENG. J. MED. 2205, 2205.

[2] Kindy, K. (2017) House GOP quietly advances key elements of tort reform, retrieved from *https://www.washingtonpost.com/national/house-gop-quietly-advances-key-elements-of-tort-reform/2017/03/09/d52213b2-0414-11e7-b1e9-a05d3c21f7cf_story.html?utm_term=.4d3c56fe7870* on July 10, 2018.

4

Campaign Contributions and Legislative Harmony

Contributions in 2000 from the insurance industry totaled $41,782,801 for federal elections, with 65 percent of those funds given to the Republicans and 34 percent to the Democrats. The amount spent for lobbyists for ederal initiatives that year was $86,975,440.[84]
– Center for Responsive Politics

The amount of campaign contributions made by the insurance industry is staggering. For example, in 2000, the insurance industry made a total of $41,782,801 in campaign contributions and spent another $86,975,440 paying lobbyists for their services during the same year.[85] This is a total of $1,287,582,410 dollars spent on insurance industry interests – all of which is funded indirectly by policyholders through premium payments and increases.

The following is a detailed chart showing the relationship between campaign contributions, the amount of money spend on lobbying, and the number of uninsured.

Year	Amount of Dollars Spent on Federal Contributions from Insurance Industry	Amount of Dollars Spent on Lobby Efforts from the Insurance Industry	Number of Uninsured Americans
2002	$37.564,920	$92,601,162	43.8 Million
2000	$41,782,801	$86,975,440	38.7 Million
1998	$30,358,554	$77,207,908	44.3 Million
1997	N/A	$65,581.955	43.4 Million

Information was provided by Center for Responsive Politics, *www.census.gov&sopr.senate.gov*

Note: These numbers represent contributions within the insurance industry from all types of insurance services.

This data reflects a steady increase in money spent in lobbying efforts between 1997 and 2002. It is important to note that the higher number of uninsureds leave the burden of rising costs on those who continue to pay for insurance. As lobbying expenses and contributions increase, the added burden of higher financial obligations relevant to these increased amounts is placed on the remaining policyholders. The public is very much aware of higher annual premiums; however, it is critical that policyholders understand that as the number of uninsureds has risen, and the amount of dollars spent on lobbying effort has increased, along with the higher premiums.

President Bush has stated that a government-run system is not the answer to solving the health care crisis even though in 2002 more than 43 million Americans did not have health care coverage.[86] In his State of the Union address on January 20, 2004, President Bush said,

> "A government-run health care system is the wrong prescription. By keeping costs under control, expanding access, and helping more Americans afford coverage, we will preserve the system of private medicine that makes America's health care the best in the world."[87]

Was President Bush's speech reflective of actual citizens' beliefs in the U.S., or was it the belief of a select group of elected officials? If the high number of uninsured is a problem in the United States, the assumption could be made that the system as we know it today clearly is not working. Is the argument against a government-run health care system founded in its potential inadequacies, or is the insurance industry itself fighting to maintain its own nucleus of gainful employment and profit by continuing to "fight the battle of health care" on the policyholders' dime?

The only answer to this question is to review data that will reveal the opinion about the health care system from the American public. Research that would answer the question as to how American citizens feel about their own health care should be compared to other countries that have government-run health care services.

According to a report by the Commonwealth Fund 2002 from a study entitled the International Health Policy Survey, 44 percent of U.S. adults with health problems reported being "not very satisfied" with their health care system – the second highest rate in the survey as compared to New Zealand (48 percent), Canada (36 percent), Australia (35 percent), and the United Kingdom (31 percent). When asked to name the two biggest problems with the U.S. health care system, nearly half (48 percent) named the high cost of health care and one-quarter named the inadequate coverage of services.[88]

It is important to note that this survey represents the opinion of those "depending on the U.S. health care system" at the time of the survey as opposed to those who believe how it will cover them when they may need it (at a future date). The critical point in this study is that many citizens may be hoodwinked into believing that once they need affordable and effective health care services, it will be available to them. However, according to the survey, reliability on affordable and patient-focused health care certainly was not the reality for a large percentage of those who were dependent on the system at the time of the survey.

One of the strongest arguments against implementing a government-run system stems from the belief that wait times for medical treatment would become excessively long. The following is the result of a survey comparing the issue of "wait times" in the United States to other countries who currently have government-run health care systems.

Difficulty Seeing a Specialist and Waiting Problems

	AUS	CAN	NZ	UK	US
Very or somewhat difficult to see a specialist.	41%	53%	36%	38%	40%

The following were "big problems" in the past two years

	AUS	CAN	NZ	UK	US
Long waits at hospitals admission.	20%	28%	21%	9%	14%
Long waits for doctor appointments.	17%	24%	5%	21%	14%
Delay of scheduled surgeryor procedure due to cancellation.	10%	16%	9%	10%	5%

*Data provided by: The Commonwealth Fund 2002 International Health Policy Survey

This data reflects that the United States has lower wait times and fewer delays in scheduled procedures; however, it is still important to note that the significance of the difference on a percentage scale is, at most, less than a maximum of 5 percent against the next country that has a government-run health care system. The American public must ask itself if a minimal increase in wait times is an acceptable "trade off" for health care.

Regulation and Legislation from a State Perspective

From a state level perspective, lobbying and political efforts have been done on a much smaller scale because the preferred objective is to seek favorable federal rules and regulation. According to *followthemoney.org*, the amount of $3,067,393 was given in 2000 for combined state-level initiatives. This is not to imply that the insurance industry does not take state initiatives lightly when it comes to states who attempt to pass legislation to impose or change regulations through legislative initiatives. These attempts are not usually met with strong industry opposition.

An example of this comes from the State of Tennessee when the Tennessee General Assembly in 2003 reportedly took aim at revising the negotiation practices of Blue Cross Blue Shield of Tennessee. In response to this action by the legislature, the insurance giant quickly added more lobbyists to their staff in late February of 2003.[89]

The Texas based political organization, Campaigns for People, acknowledged the hot button issue of insurance is yet another reason why the group believes Texas needs stronger campaign finance disclosure rules. A report from this organization shows campaign contributions from the insurance industry to legislative candidates are slated to increase by 25 percent from the 2000 election cycle in Texas. The group said that from June 2001 to June 2002, the industry gave $300,628 in contributions. Based on the industry's pattern of giving from the 2000 election, that figure is expected to grow to about $677,000 through the next election. "The insurance industry's two-prong strategy of campaign contributions and lobbyists has shown proficient ability to defeat or water down many significant consumer reforms,: according to Dietrich Knabe from Campaigns for People.[90]

In 2003, a report released by mental health and government reform advocates in New York revealed that the insurance industry's lobbying expenses, campaign contributions and six to seven figure salaries for top officials are contributing to the rising cost of health care in that state. Health insurers routinely fight state mandates for new services, claiming they force health care premiums to rise. But the report found 14 insurance companies in New York together spent $1.5 million on lobbying and campaign contributions in 2002 and had an average CEO salary of $826,888 – roughly two-and-a-half times the $312,778 average New York CEO's pay in other industries.[91]

According the data in this chapter regarding political contributions and lobbying efforts we note that between 2002 (page 42) and 2015 there was a significant increase in the amount of an increase of $71.5 million. The lobbying efforts increased between 2000 (page 42) to 2016 in the amount of $46.5 million. In 2016, the highest year for political contributions dollars, it was also the year of the largest annual increase of insurance premiums.

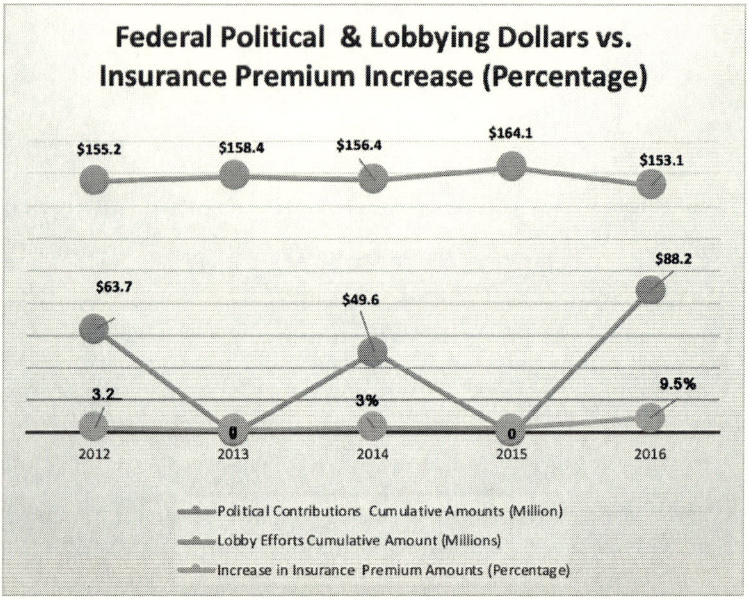

& https://www.kff.org/health-reform/fact-sheet/analysis-of-2016-premium-changes-in-the-affordable-care-acts-health-insurance-marketplaces/
Retrieved August 18, 2018.

5

Medical Bills and Bankruptcy

A record number of Americans file into U.S. Bankruptcy Court as morepeople are being pushed over the edge by their unpaid medical bills.
— *The Boston Globe,* July 19, 2003

This idea of "pay premiums and get coverage" is far from a reality for many. According to *Smart Money* magazine, more Americans filed for bankruptcy in 2003 than ever before. There was a record 1.6 million personal bankruptcies filed in 2003. That is just a bit less than double the 812,898 bankruptcies filed in 1993. Broken down into another perspective, that is one bankruptcy for every 73 American households, or one bankruptcy filed every 20 seconds, according to the American Bankruptcy Institute.[92] And the reason the number is currently so high is because unpaid health care bills are now the leading cause of personal bankruptcy in the United States.[93]

The consequences associated with rising health care costs extend beyond the reach of individuals and families who default on their medical bills to impact society in numerous ways. The public is forced to foot the bill on bankruptcy through the higher payment of goods and services to cover the losses of businesses that are financially strapped when their customers file bankruptcy. The health of our society is threatened when health care services are not affordable to those who need it – thereby negatively impacting the productivity of American workers.

The History of Bankruptcy

Even though the United States is experiencing record numbers of bankruptcy filings, the actual process of bankruptcy has been in existence for centuries. The origins of bankruptcy have been accurately described by Greta Schneider, economist, writer, and speaker, in her book entitled *Holistic Bankruptcy* published in 1998. This section reviews Ms. Schneider's research on the history of bankruptcy.

The origin of the word 'bankrupt' is Italian and comes from banca rota, which means bench broken. This refers to the medieval Italian banking system where bankers and money lenders operated from benches on wide boulevards. When they ran out of money and their operations failed, the authorities stopped their businesses by physically breaking and destroying their benches. A similar definition exists from the Latin, *banca rupta*, which means bank broken.

Bankruptcy has a long and tumultuous history. From the royal houses and privileged aristocracies of Europe to sea captains, country gentry and simple farmers of past centuries, to the average rural/ urban/suburban dwellers of today, people from every walk of life have stared into the eye of the storm called *debt*. Bankruptcy existed as early as the sixteenth century in colonial America following the passage of the first British bankruptcy law in 1543. Any person who couldn't repay debt would be imprisoned for as long as their creditors could pay the cost of their imprisonment.

Individual American colonies maintained their own bankruptcy rules. Some colonies were more lenient towards debtors than others. One such bankruptcy haven was the Georgia colony because it gave debtors fairer treatment compared to other colonies. A statute passed in the Georgia colonial legislature discharged (cancelled) debts to give debtors a fresh start.

The New York colony made creditors pay three shillings a week (approximately 36 cents) to keep a defaulting debtor in prison. The Virginia colony passed a law in the early 1700's that a defaulting debtor could not be jailed for more than 20 days. The debtor was taken to court and swore under oath that he was unable to pay his debts. All of the debtor's property *except* for the clothes on his back and his work supplies were seized. After serving the 20-day sentence the debtor was released from both jail and the obligation to repay his debts.

Debtors' existence was also remembered in the United States Constitution. In 1789 the founding fathers included debtors in Article I, Section 8, Clause 4, giving Congress the power *"to establish uniform laws on the subject of bankruptcies throughout the United States."*

Bankruptcy became an official part of American law in 1841 when the discharge of debts (cancellation) was recognized. The first modern American bankruptcy law was called "The National Bankruptcy Act." Under this 1898 law, the emphasis was on a fair distribution of assets to creditors; helping debtors free themselves of debt was only a secondary consideration. This law called bankruptcy filers "bankrupts" and those who administered estates the "receivers." Cases were often heard by a "referee in bankruptcy" and the final decision rested with the bankruptcy court.

A number of changes occurred in the twentieth century because the country was deep in an economic depression in the early 1930's. With 1933 marking the beginning of the "New Deal" under President Franklin Delano Roosevelt, a new consciousness arose and became a political issue. This was the recognition of the plight of the rural and urban poor. Congress acted and reformed the bankruptcy process by amending the National Bankruptcy Act to shift emphasis towards giving debtors a fresh start, and secondarily ensuring that creditors were given fair distribution of residual assets. In an effort to accommodate the changing social and economic circumstances, amendments to bankruptcy laws of the 1930's are continually being added.[94]

The "At Risk" Group for Bankruptcy

According to a survey by the Center for Financing, Access and Cost Trends, the average annual health insurance premium in 2000 for a single person enrolled in an employee insurance program was $2,655 and $6,772 for families.[95]

As employers continue to reduce benefits, or pass their increases onto employees directly, the question becomes, *who is most vulnerable to be impacted by rising insurance costs?*

The following represents the average median weekly earnings of workers and the ethnic percentage of the entire U.S. population and uninsured individuals.

	Median Weekly Earnings	% of Total Pop.	% of Uninsured (under age 65)
Caucasian	$591	75.1%	15.2%
Black/African American	$468	12.3%	20.0%
Hispanic/Latino	$396	12.5%	35.0%

2000 Census Information.[96]

Median weekly earnings information is from the report entitled "Counting Minorities: A Brief History and a Look at the Future."[97]

Information regarding the percentage of uninsured was provided by the report "Health, United States, 2000 Table 129."[98]

Findings for all categories for other specific ethnic groups are not available.

This information reveals that lower income directly impacts the percentage of uninsured in a particular ethnic category. Today the highest numbers of bankruptcy filers are single women (of all ethnic backgrounds), African Americans, and Hispanic homeowners. These groups are 500 percent more likely to file bankruptcy compared to white (two incomes and/or with a white male as head of the household) homeowners.[99] Congresswoman Stephanie Tubbs Jones commented on recent economic data,

> "This economy has had a disproportionate affect on minorities in this country, particularly African

> Americans. According to the U.S. Courts Administrative Office's bankruptcy statistics, 1,625,208 households filed for bankruptcy in 2003, a 33 percent increase from 2000. That is nearly one bankruptcy every 19 seconds. For minorities, the statistics are even worse. According to an article by Elizabeth Warren and Amelia Warren Tyagi entitled *The Two Income Trap*, African Americans and Hispanics are much more likely to go bankrupt. Hispanic homeowners are nearly three times more likely than white homeowners to file for bankruptcy, and black homeowners are nearly six times more likely than white homeowners."[100]

The single largest group of bankruptcy filers are households headed by women. They account for 40 percent of bankruptcies because women are often unable to collect child support money they are owed from former spouses or partners.[101] This problem is further exacerbated by the significant difference in earning potential between women and men.

According to a study by the Institute for Women's Policy Research, women, on the average, earn 76 cents for every dollar earned by a man. Hispanic women suffer most from pay disparities, earning only 52.5 cents for every dollar earned by white men. Overall, women from all racial and ethnic backgrounds earned 67.5 cents for every dollar earned by a white man.[102]

The fastest growing group of bankruptcy filers is the elderly population. A report done by the Consumer Bankruptcy Project at Harvard University found that about 82,000

American over 65 years of age filed for bankruptcy in 2001, which is up 244 percent since 1991.[103] Some experts believe that overwhelming rising medical expenses are the culprit as Social Security and pension checks don't stretch as far as needed.

In addition to higher health care costs, seniors often receive less Social Security income when a spouse dies. Many retirees have also seen companies cut back their pensions and health care coverage, leaving them to reach further into their dwindling savings accounts to cover the differences.[104] Once these funds are depleted, the only other alternative is for them to file bankruptcy.

Houston-based personal bankruptcy trustee Ben B. Floyd says that he is now seeing (retired) people who "obviously had a white-collar background come in looking lost." Personal bankruptcy lawyers across the country say they have witnessed a tidal shift in their practices, seeing older clients with long work histories. "These people didn't take their credit cards to Atlantic City," says Gabriel Del Virginia, a New York bankruptcy attorney. "It's largely because people lost their jobs or had a catastrophic illness."[105]

In the U.S. we continue to see a large number of bankruptcies due to medical bills. As noted in this chapter, such legal action due to medical bills continue to plague the nation across different age groups. In comparison to other nations such as Britain, France, Japan, Germany, Canada, the Netherlands and Switzerland, all of these nations have not had any bankruptcy filings, compared to the U.S. where there are approximately 643,000 (average) filings per year.[1]

The follow chart reflects the age and number of bankruptcies filed in the U.S. that were directly tied to medical expenses in 2013.

Medical Bankruptcy by Age

Age Range	% of Total Bankruptcies 2013, Estimated	US Medical-Related Bankruptcies 2013, Estimated	Size of Household	People Living in Households with medical-Related Bankruptcy 2013, Estimated
18-24	2.3%	14,618	2.41	35,229
25-34	18.7%	120,708	2.86	344,622
35-44	28.9%	186,812	3.35	624,888
45-54	26.4%	170,875	2.81	480,159
55-64	15.8%	102,080	2.18	222,534
65+	8.0%	51,719	1.76	90,767

Source: NerdWallet Health Analysis

https://www.snopes.com/fact-check/643000-bankruptcies-in-the-u-s-every-year-due-to-medical-bills/
Retrieved December 12, 2018

6

China and Vietnam: Progressive Economies Make Health Care a Priority

In the search to find a solution to help the failing American health care system, a review of foreign programs reveal that China and Vietnam, two of the fastest growing economies in the world, are taking pro-active steps to improve their health and medical programs for their citizens. To support the demands of their expanding economic status, the governments of both countries are making health care a priority. They know that a healthy work force will be able to accommodate the demand for employment.

Today China has the fastest growing economy in the world.[106] With their rapid economic development and the improvement of their standard of living, China's health care industry experienced rapid growth over the last decade. Access to health care facilities and treatment is readily available to the population as more hospitals have been built and the number of doctors practicing medicine has steadily risen since 1991.[107]

Vietnam's growth rate during 2003 was approximately 7 percent, making the country the fastest growing economy after China.[108] In 2004, the Socialist Republic of Vietnam received a loan from the Asian Development Bank and a grant from the Government of Sweden through the Swedish International Development Cooperation Agency to improve health care services in Vietnam, especially for the poor and disadvantaged population located in rural and remote areas. The specific objectives for the use of the funds are to:

1) improve the availability of and access to quality health services, especially for the poor and disadvantaged,
2) improve affordability and utilization of health services, especially for the poor, and
3) strengthen the capacity of the health system to address effectively the health needs of the people.[109]

Rapid economic growth in Vietnam has already reduced the percentage of poverty from 58 percent in 1993 to 29 percent in 2002.[110] The plan to improve health care is designed to cut the poverty level even more because healthy workers will be able to increase their annual earnings and improve their social economic class. The Vietnamese government has been committed to upgrading facilities and equipment to improve the quality of health care services, to expand the preventative health infrastructure, and to add more social disease centers.

In addition to providing funding for new training, there is a priority on human resources development through enhancing the skills of health care service providers by training activities and strengthening the educational content at secondary medical schools. Government officials are dedicated to strengthening the financing and management of the system by supporting the effective implementation of the new health care initiative to grow an even stronger economy.[111]

Franco-Vietnamese Hospital: Foreign Investment Helps Solve Health Care Problems

Over the years the Vietnamese government has believed the solution to health care for its citizens is through a national health insurance system. A National Health Insurance Board was created in 1992 with the task of offering an insurance system for all industrial workers and government employees. Premium levels were set low at 3 percent, with employers covering 2 percent of the costs and employees contributing 1 percent from their pay checks. The system provides access to health care treatment and services to state-run facilities.

Because the system has benefited those who previously did not have access to health care services, ongoing problems have plagued the success of the program. One of the main complaints about the system is that low quality service is being provided and, in many cases, insurance does not cover the cost of treatment. Many patients are opting to pay for their own care even if they have insurance. Hospital administrators claim that the insurance fund rarely pays for services, and when they are reimbursed, they only receive a fraction of what is owed to them. The situation has escalated since the inception of the national health insurance system because many hospitals refuse to accept insurance cards presented by patients and instead demand cash payment upfront.

A 1997 report issued by the Vietnam government proposed solutions to improve the health care situation. The proposals included a variety of diverse forms of ownerships of health care facilities that included semi-public hospitals, joint-venture hospitals, and private hospitals that includes those owned 100 percent by foreign investors.[112]

Under the Vietnamese government's incentive to attract foreign investors, a group of French doctors decided to take advantage of the opportunity to improve health care in Vietnam by building the Franco-Vietnamese Hospital (FV). The hospital, which opened in 2003, is centrally located in Saigon South near Ho Chi Minh City. The six level, 230 bed facility required an investment of approximately 40 million (US) dollars to build, and offers a variety of medical services using state-of-the-art medical technology.[113] The medical staff has 18 full-time French doctors, 25 full-time Vietnamese doctors, and a staff providing expertise in 26 medical and surgical specialties. The hospital's mission is to provide international quality health care at affordable prices to the people of Vietnam. In an effort to promote health wellness and encourage patients to seek preventive care options and annual check-ups, the hospital offers a membership program for $1500 (US dollars) that includes:

- Priority reception and check-in.
- Unlimited free consultations in selected specialties.
- 1 free annual health screening.
- 1 free annual dental cleaning.
- 1 free annual ophthalmology screening.
- 10 percent discount on selected investigative procedures.
- 5 percent discount on private rooms.
- Complimentary transportation.
- Bi-monthly FV Hospital newsletter.
- Check-up reminders.
- Visiting doctors' schedules.
- New member welcome pack.[114]

This foreign investment has proven so successful that within one year of its opening the hospital reached its breakeven point. FV general director, Dr. Jean-Marcel Guillon stated, "We've made the right decision to invest in Vietnam where there is a demand for international hospitals changing reasonable fees."[115] The success of this hospital clearly represents the success of government initiatives to promote foreign investment in Vietnam's health care industry.

7

Conclusion: Pick Your Buddy – Insurance Companies or Government?

"As we enter 2003, Travelers holds a solid market position, has astrong balance sheet and has significant earnings potential," commented Mr. Robert Lipp, CEO of Travelers' Casualty & Surety Company.[116]
— *Insurance Day,* January 27, 2003

The American health care system is systematically following a similar path that France encountered in the eighteenth century that contributed to the French Revolution. While the insurance industry profits soar, the growing number of uninsured is creating a bigger gap between the "have's" and "have not's" as many families are simply unable to afford coverage. It is reasonable to expect that at some point all citizens will incur an unexpected injury or illness that will require medical attention. This creates the issue of inevitable medical expenses, and combined with minimal or no insurance, may end up forcing patients to file bankruptcy, which ultimately hurts our society in many ways.

In some of my previously published articles I recommended more regulation for the insurance industry as a method of controlling them. I have since changed my opinion and I now believe that with the level of political power of the insurance industry (from their campaign contributions and lobbying efforts), more regulation would be pointless. New regulation may be an effective short-term fix of the problem, but there is no doubt that once the new regulatory playing field was established, the insurance industry's lobbying efforts would immediately begin to work to change those laws back to more favorable ones for themselves. And with time and the money they have to spend, they would be successful, thereby negating any progress made in tightening the regulatory rules.

A government-run social medical system that benefits everyone is the only way to create a society of healthy citizens. This is not to say that any socialized plan will be perfect. Improving and reevaluating a socialized system will need to be a priority during each legislative session.

There are three immediate changes needed in the American health care system before a positive shift in the delivery of quality care is accomplished. First, a health care system that provides equal services for all citizens is the only way to establish full participation that will create a health society at manageable costs. The more people using the health care system, the lower the per-patient costs paid by each individual through their taxes and contributions to the health care system. By eliminating insurance premiums and other costs controlled by insurance and drug companies today, the cost shift to higher taxes will in the end result in more savings to each citizen because the payee base is larger and controlled by government.

Second, similar to the privately run Franco-Vietnamese hospital in Saigon, providing investment and financial incentives for doctors to establish their own health care facilities and services without excessive government regulation that under today's status may be tainted with pro-insurance industry incentives resulting from lobby efforts, would benefit those who want private health care options.

This opportunity creates a new market for private health care services run by doctors that takes off the handcuffs of insurance industry pricing contracts that reduces their fees. In addition to making less money under these contracts, doctors are confronted each year with rising malpractice insurance premiums that are driving many of America's finest doctors out of the profession. Allowing doctors to engage in their practices with more flexibility over pricing structure of services ultimately lowers administrative costs now spent on handling extensive insurance documentation. This arrangement may only benefit doctors and patients who seek private care.

And lastly, to make the new system work, American government lawmakers must make health care a priority. The proper reviews of a government system need to take place annually to identify areas that need to be changed and improved, as clearly this will be a new arena for all of us. If we ignore our health care demand for even a brief moment we are risking the possibility of hurting future generations who depend on us to create and maintain a healthy population. For those lawmakers who choose to ignore health care issues as a priority in their agendas, it is easier to elect new government officials when necessary compared to attempting to re-regulate or change the insurance industry during each legislative session.

Personally, I believe the optimal situation for the United States would be to have an entire system run by doctors alone. However, with high unemployment and with many of our citizens in a desperate financial crisis, this would lead to a system where, like in pre-revolution France, many would simply not seek medical treatment because the costs would make such services prohibitive. A plan of this nature at this point in American history, is simply not feasible.

Another issue to consider: From the viewpoint of someone who hasn't yet entered retirement, I would rather pay a higher tax and spread the risk among a large population pool who would share the entire costs, then risk having the ongoing runaway premium expenses that we are seeing today continue on into the future. Those of us in the work force today simply cannot plan for our retirement with the large fluctuations in medical expense that we are seeing today. Without government control of the health care system, the insurance industry will continue to offer menial changes here and there, but ultimately profit and political power will always be the driving force behind their agenda.

In review of health care since the first edition of this book was published, the enactment of the Affordable Care Act (Obamacare) in 2010 significantly changed the American health care system. As it continues to be a contentious issue between political parties, it did succeed in providing health care cover to more than 20 million Americans. Additionally, it has provided more financial security by avoiding the often catastrophic result of financial stress, and possibly bankruptcy, due to a lack coverage or non-coverage when a medical event occurs. Furthermore, it reduced the inequality of coverage whereby income levels determine premium amounts without the compromise of benefits that has been typically much less for low wage earners. Obamacare also requires services to be provided by insurance companies and it no longer caps the amount that an insurer will pay. Because of this mandate, patients now have access to what they need without the worry of being cut off from benefits an insurance company. Finally, Obamacare has been created to save more than it costs from a mix of spending and taxes along with cuts to other programs, therefore it is expected to save federal dollars at least until 2025.[1]

1 Sanger-Katz, M. (2017). Grading Obamas success, failures and incompletes. Retrieved December 12, 2018, from *https://www.nytimes.com/2017/02/05/upshot/grading-obamacare-successes-failures-and-incompletes.html*

About the Author

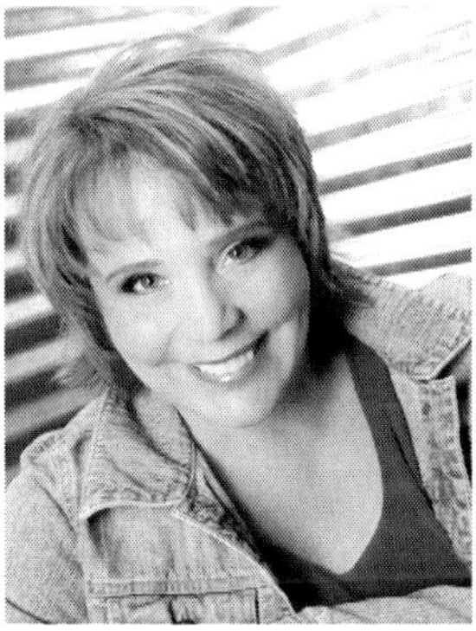

Dr. René Ryman is an Assistant Professor at the American University of Paris who teaches International Business courses to graduate and undergraduate students. Her research includes the understanding of cultures from the perspective of economic and historic development that incorporates regional and community evolution toward modern day success stemming from public policy. Dr. Ryman is committed to sharing her understanding of how commerce has played a significant role in the sustainability of cultures throughout the world and patterns of changes in the environment that help or hindered economic progression throughout the centuries.

Dr. Ryman resides in Paris, France, and her educational background includes completing her post-doctorate studies in AACSB certification at the University of Southern California and her doctorate degree at the University of Sarasota/ Argosy. She holds a Master's in International Studies from the University of Denver, an M.B.A. from the Lake Forest Graduate School of Management and a B.S. degree from Elmhurst College.

Note to Readers

Thank you for reading my book. I sincerely hope you enjoyed reading it as much as I enjoyed researching and writing it.

I am now in the process of starting my next book, which will cover individual cases of people who have accepted settlement offers that have now left them in a financial bind due to their inability to pay their medical bills. If you or someone you know is in this situation, I would like to hear your story. I am also interested in stories from people who were involved in personal injuries cases where the defense attorney used unethical and illegal threats and tactics, such as questioning during depositions about unrelated topics to an accident to scare, deter or embarrass a plaintiff from seeking justice. If you would like to share your story, or if you know someone who would like to discuss their situation with me, please email me at *rene_ryman@msn.com.*

It is my hope that awareness and public disclosure will start to turn the system toward a positive future for our society.

References

1 Diane Levick, "Traveler's Earnings Up 33%," *The Hartford Courant*, July 18, 2003, Sec. Business, p. E2.

2 Tony Pugh, "Ranks of American Uninsured Swells to 41 Million," *Knight Ridder Washington Bureau*, September 29, 2002.

3 Michael Perrault, "PacifiCare Threatens to Dump Small Groups Major Health Insurer Demands State Pass Regulatory Reforms," *Rocky Mountain News*, March 2, 2001.

4 David Pilla, "Conseco to Shut Down Remaining Health Businesses" *Best Week*, February 18, 2002.

5 Julie Piotrowski, "How Secure is the Safety Net?" *Modern Healthcare*, February 25, 2002,
<*http://www.ncbi.nlm.nih.gov/entrez/query.fcgi?db=pubmed &cmd=Display& dopt=pubmed_pubmed&from_uid= 11913040* >
accessed October 31, 2004.

6 Michael Lasalandra, "Nearly Half in U.S. Claim Problem with Health Care," *The Boston Herald*, August 31, 2001, Sec. News, p. 20.

7 Robert A. Clifford, "Defining Bad Faith," Chicago Lawyer, October 1, 2000, < *http:// www.cliffordlaw.com/press/ detail.aspx?prssrmID=000000235100* >
accessed October 31, 2004.

8 Brook Raflo, “Face to Face with Reimbursement,” *PRIMEDIA Business Magazine,* August 1, 2003, <*http://homecaremag.com/mag/medical_face_face_reimbursement /index.html*> accessed on October 31, 2004.

9 Todd Richmond, “Review Panel Reverses 42 Percent of Health Insurance Decisions,” *The Associated State and Local Press*, June 11, 2003.

10 Kevin M. Quinley, “Boot Me Up C3P0. Assessing Claim Evaluation Software, Meet Your New Risk Manager R2D2,” *Claims Magazine*, July, 2002, <*http://www.claimsmag.com/Issues/July02/risk_management.asp*> accessed October 31, 2004.

11 Candace Heckman, “Insurers’ Use of Colossus, A Service to Judge the Worth of Claims, Comes Under Fire: Does Company ‘Low-Ball’ Pain?” *Seattle Post-Intelligencer*, May 15, 2003, < *http://static.highbeam.com/s/seattlepostintelligencerseattlewa /may152003/insurersuseofcolossusaservicetojudgetheworthofclaims/*> accessed October 31, 2004.

12 “Basic Injury Values for Bad Faith Cases,” *The Jury Verdict Research, Series No. 6.80.1.*

13 Rene Ryman, “Insurance Company Bad Faith: The Real Culprit Responsible for Rising Insurance Premiums,” *Trial Talk*, Feb/March, 2003.

14 Matthais Rieker, “Seeing Sector Rebound, Street Bullish on Travelers,” *The American Banker*, April 25, 2002, <*www.americanbanker.com*> accessed October 1, 2004.

15 Centers for Medicare and Medicaid Services, "Health Care Spending Reaches $1.6 Trillion in 2002," <*www. cms.hhs.gov*> accessed October 1, 2004.

16 Insurance Finder, "Insurance Information," <*http://www.insurancefinder.com/other/insurancehistory.html*> accessed October 1, 2004.

17 Wikipedia, The Free Encyclopedia, "History of Insurance," < *http://en.wikipedia.org /wiki/Insurance#History_of_ insurance*> accessed October 1, 2004.

18 Insurance Finder, supra.

19 Wikipedia, supra.

20 Tufts Managed Care Institute, "*A Brief History of Managed Care,*" 1998, p 1.

21 A. E. Radich, "*A Brief History of the Healthcare Industry in America,*" Ohio State College of Osteopathic Medicine, <*http://www.ooanet.org/pdf/OUCOMManagedCare .pdf*> accessed October 1, 2004.

22 Tufts, supra, pp. 1-2.

23 Radich, supra, p. 3.

24 Janet L. Lerman, "*Medical Practice Strategies: Managed Care-Business Laws,*" <*http://www.medicalpracticecme.com/Class%201/Articles%20for%20class%201 /article1class1.htm*> accessed October 1, 2004, p. 5.

25 New Labor Forum, 2004 Summer, Vol. 13, #2, <*www.qcpages.qc.edu /newlaborforum*> accessed October 1, 2004.

26 Tufts, supra, p. 4.

27 Lerman, supra, p. 6.

28 Ibid, p. 7.

29 "Paul Ellwood and the Genesis of Managed Health Care," *The Burton Report*, <*http://www.burtonreport.com/infhealthcare/managedellwood.htm*> accessed October 1, 2004.

30 "Medicare May Go Bust by 2019," *CNN Money*, March 23, 2004, <*http://money.cnn .com/2004/03/23/news/economy/medicare/*> accessed October 1, 2004.

31 Statistical Section Centers of Medicare and Medicaid website, <,*www.cms.hhs.gov /statistics*> accessed October 1, 2004.

32 U. S. Census Bureau, *Income, Poverty, and Health Insurance Coverage in the United States: 2003,* U. S. Department of Commerce, August 2004, p. 14, <*http://www.census .gov/prod/2004pubs/p60-226.pdf*> accessed October 1, 2004.

33 Alan Forest, *The French Revolution and the Poor*, St. Martin's Press, New York, 1981, p. 60. (Forest's book describes French health care reform under Emperor

Napoleon Bonaparte, who assumed power in 1791 after the French Revolution.)

34 Laurence Brockliss and Colin Jones, *The Medical World of Early Modern France*, Clarendon Press, Oxford, UK, 1997, p. 80.

35 Ibid, p. 62.

36 Forest, supra, p. 34.

37 Ibid, p. 35.

38 Ibid, p. 278.

39 Matthew Ramsey, *Professional and Popular Medicine in France*, 1770–1830, Cambridge University Press, Cambridge, UK, 1988, p. 62.

40 Ibid, p. 62.

41 Ibid.

42 Forest, supra, pp. 36-38.

43 Ibid, p. 44.

44 Ibid, p. 40.

45 Ibid, p. 43.

46 Brockliss and Jones, supra, p. 802.

47 Evelyn B. Ackerman, *Health Care in the Parisian Countryside*, 1800–1914, Rutgers University Press, Rutgers, NJ, 1990, p. 60.

48 Forest, supra, p. 40.

49 Brockliss and Jones, supra, p. 803.

50 Pugh, supra. 51 Lee Murphy, "Workers Drop Out of Coverage: Higher Costs Price More Employees Out of the Market," *Crain's Chicago Business*, August 6, 2001.

52 Larry Lipman, "Health Insurance 'Perfect Storm' Will Soak Workers," *Seattle Post Intelligencer*, <*www.seattlepi.nwsource.com/business.com*> accessed July 1, 2004.

53 Pugh, supra.

54 Murphy, supra.

55 Karen Kirchgasser, "2 Million Americans Lost Their Health Insurance in 2001, the Largest One-Year Increase in Nearly a Decade," *PR Newswire*, February 12, 2002, <*www.prnewswire.com*> accessed October 31, 2004.

56 Andy Miller, "Study Says Increase in Premiums May Leave 200,000 Georgia Residents Uninsured," *Atlanta Journal and Constitution*, March 9, 2001.

57 Murphy, supra.

58 Piotrowski, supra.

59 Perrault, supra, Bus. Sec. p. 9B.

60 Matt Brady, "Northeast Zone: R.I. Exodus Continues," *Insurance Chronicle*, April 22, 2002.

61 David Pilla, "Conseco to Shut Down Remaining Health Businesses," *Best Wire*, February 14, 2002.

62 Ibid.

63 Arizona, California, Colorado, South Dakota, Connecticut, Idaho, Washington, Texas, Utah, Arkansas, Delaware, Illinois, Iowa, Kansas, Massachusetts, Minnesota, New Hampshire, Oregon, Vermont and Wisconsin.

64"HRSA Press Office, Nine More States Receive HHS Grants to Develop Plans Extending Health Insurance Coverage to All Citizens," *U.S. Newswire*, February 27, 2001.

65 Brad Smith, "EDS Signs $100 Million in Government Health Care Business," *Canada News Wire*, September 25, 2002.

66 David Himmelstein, "Health Spending in U.S. Is Higher Than Any Other Nation: Americans Pay For National Health Insurance But Don't Get It." *Ascribe Newswire*, July 8, 2002.

67 Himmelstein, ibid.

68 C. Hundley, "No End Seen in Rising Premiums," *St. Petersburg Times*, September 7, 2002.

69 U. S. Department of Labor, Bureau of Labor Statistics, *<http://www.bls.gov/news.release/cpi.toc.htm>* accessed October 1, 2004.

70 J. Gavin, "Liability Lawsuits Rise Despite Bevy of Reforms, Colo. Restrictions Have Minimal Impact," *Denver Post*, March 1, 1992.

71 M. Ogborn, "Insurance Industry Invents Another Hoax," *Denver Post*, November 20, 1989.

72 Michael Perrault, "Going Up: State Farm to Raise Car Rates an Average of 10% in Oct.," *Rocky Mountain News*, September 5, 2002, Bus. Sec. p. 1B.

73 Gavin, supra, p. A1.

74 Ogborn, supra, p. C2. 75 J. Wojcik, "Dispute Over Bad Faith a Matter of Perspective," *Business Insurance*, Vol. 30, Issue 19, p. 15, 1996.

76 State Farm Mutual Automobile Insurance Co. v. Campbell, No. 01-1289, (U.S.S.CT., argued December 11, 2002).

77 Wojcik, supra, p. 15.

78 Ibid.

79 Ibid.

80 Robert A. Clifford, "Defining Bad Faith," *Chicago Lawyer*, October 1, 2000, < *http://www.cliffordlaw.com/press/detail.aspx?prssrmID=000000235100*> accessed October 31, 2004.

81 J. Kelso and K. Kelso, *Jury Verdicts in Insurance Bad Faith Cases*, Institute for Legislative Practice, McGeorge School of Law, University of the Pacific, 1996.

82 "Basic Injury Values for Bad Faith Cases," *The Jury Verdict Research, Series No. 6.80.1.*

83 Kelso, supra.

84 <*http://www.opensecrets.org/industries/indus.asp?Ind=F09*> accessed July 15, 2004.

85 <*http://www.opensecrets.org/industries/indus.asp?Ind=F09*> accessed May 1, 2004.

86 U. S. Census Bureau, Health Insurance Coverage in the United States: 2002, issued September 2003, *Consumer Income*, U. S. Department of Commerce, <*http://www .census.gov/prod/2003pubs/p60-223.pdf* > accessed May 1, 2004.

87 <*www.whitehouse.gov*> accessed May 1, 2004.

88 Commonwealth Fund, 2002 International Health Survey, *The United States Health Care Systems: Views and Experiences of Adults with Health Problems*, Publication 644, May 2003.

89 A. M. Heher, "HCA, Blue Cross Hire More Lobbyists," *Chattanooga Time Free Press*, March 6, 2003, p. A1.

90 N. Gott, "Group Releases Contribution Report from Insurers," *The Associated State and Free Press*, Austin, TX, October 8, 2002.

91 E. Benjamin, "Groups Hit Health Insurers on Spending: Albany CEO Salaries, Lobbying and Political Contributions Drive Up Costs Consumer Advocates Say," *The Times Union*, Albany, NY, December 9, 2003, p. B3.

92 P. McGann, "Guess What Drove Bankruptcies to a New High?" *Lewiston Morning Tribune*, Idaho, June 6, 2004, p. 8A.

93 W. Point, "Skyrocketing Costs; United States' Health Care System Is Entering a Crisis," *Charleston Gazette*, West Virginia, July 21, 2003, p. 5A.

94 G. Schneider, *Holistic Bankruptcy*, Schneider Consulting Group, New York, pg. 3-4.

95 J. Branscome, "State Differences in the Cost of Job-Related Health Insurance 2000," <*www.meps.ahcpr.gov*> accessed September 20, 2004.

96 U. S. Census Bureau 2000 Census Report, *Counting Minorities: A Brief History and a Look at the Future*, <*www.census.gov*> accessed September 20, 2004.

97 U. S. Department of Labor Bureau of Labor Statistics, *Health, United States, 2000,* Table 129, pg. 24, <*www.stats.bls.gov*> accessed September 20, 2004.

98 U. S. Department of Health and Human Services, Centers for Disease Control and Prevention, *Health, United States 2000*, Table 129, p. 331, <*www.cdc.gov*> accessed September 20, 2004.

99 Consumer Federation of America Report, *Creditor-Friendly Bankruptcy Agreement That Hurts Vulnerable Debtors on the Brink of Becoming*, dated 8/28/02, <*http://www. consumerfed.org/bankruptcy_conference_agreement_4-02PDF*> accessed September 20, 2004.

100 Elizabeth Warren and Amelia Warren Tyagi, "The Two Income Trap," *Unity First Online and African American Newswire*, <*www.unityfirst.com*> accessed September 10, 2004.

101 Consumer Federation of America Report, supra.

102 P. Brogan, "Despite Progress, Women Still Trail Men in Earning Power," *Gannett News Service*, April 20, 2004.

103 Consumer Federation of America Report, supra.

104 E. A. Powell, "Debt, Bankruptcy Stalking the Elderly," *Associated Press*, July 8, 2004.

105 S. Hwang, "As Bankruptcy Filings Go Up, So Does the Age of Those Who File," *Charleston Gazette*, August 8, 2004, p. 5E.

106 J. Graham, "China's Rapid Economic Growth Raises Some Overheating Fears," *Investor's Daily,* March 16, 2004. Sec. A, Nat'l. Ed., p. A01.

107 Asia Market Information and Development Company Report, *Health Care Industry Outputs and Forecasts, Chinese Markets for Health Care*, October, 2002, pg. 1-2.

108 Asia Pulse Report, *Vietnam's GDP Growth Likely to Hit 7% This Year: World Bank*, October 22, 2003.

109 Asia Pulse Report, *ADB UN Procurement – Vietnam, Health Care System Consultants,* July 6, 2004.

110 Asia Pulse Report, October 22, 2003. supra, p. 3.

111 Asia Pulse Report, July 6, 2004, supra, p. 2.

112 International Medical Consultants Limited, *The Franco Vietnamese Hospital of Ho Chi Minh City*, Information Memorandum, January 2001, p. 20.

113 "Health and Environment: Franco-Vietnamese Hospital Set To Open In March," *Saigon Times Daily*, February 19, 2003, p. 2.

114 Franco-Vietnamese Hospital, <*www.fvhospital.com*> accessed September 20, 2004.

115 T. Ngoc, "Hospital Reaches Breakeven Point," *Saigon Times Daily*, May 14, 2003.

116 "Travelers Warns Rate Increase Will Level Off for Direct Market," *Insurance Day,* January 27, 2003.

Recommended Health Care Reading Resources

1. *An Introduction to the Health Care Crisis in America: How Did We Get Here?* Author: Stephanie Kelton, PhD. http://www.cfeps.org/health/chapters/pdf/Chapter%201%20Introduction.pdf

2. *An Introduction to Health Insurance: What Should a Consumer Know?* Author: Carol Rapaport, PhD, MSc, BSc. https://fas.org/sgp/crs/misc/R44014.pdf

3. *An introduction to medical statistics for health care professionals: Describing and presenting data.* Author: Elaine Thomas. https://onlinelibrary.wiley.com/doi/pdf/10.1002/msc.73

4. *An Introduction to Quality Assurance in Health Care.* Author: Michael Perides. https://academic.oup.com/intqhc/article/15/4/357/1793013

5. *American Health Care in Crisis: Fundamentals of Health Care Reform.* Author: Leslie Mukau, MD. http://aapsus.org/articles/38.pdf

6. Health Care Workforce Distribution and Shortage Issues in Rural America. Policy Paper. https://www.ruralhealth-

web.org/getattachment/Advocate/Policy-Documents/HealthCareWorkforceDistributionandShortageJanuary2012.pdf.aspx?lang=en-US

7. *United States Health Care Reform Progress to Date and Next Steps*. Author. B. Obama. https://jamanetwork.com/journals/jama/fullarticle/2533698

8. *The Top 10 Issues for Rural Health Care Reform.* Author: Jon Bailey. http://files.cfra.org/pdf/Ten-Rural-Issues-for-Health-Care-Reform.pdf

9. *Health Care: Issues Impacting Cost and Coverage.* Author: Aviva Aron-Dine. https://www.cbpp.org/health/health-care-issues-impacting-cost-and-coverage

10. *The Biggest U.S. Health Care Challenges Are Management Challenges.* Author: Paul Merrild. https://hbr.org/2015/02/the-biggest-u-s-health-care-challenges-are-management-challenges

11. *Health Care Around the World.* Author: Anup Shah. http://www.globalissues.org/article/774/health-care-around-the-world

12. *The Importance of Ethics In The Health Care System.* Author: Shehnaz A. Sheikh. https://www.researchgate.net/publication/268184916_The_importance_of_ethics_in_health_care_system

13. *Issues Affecting the Health of Older Citizens: Meeting the Challenge.* Authors: Jill A. Bennett, PhD, RN, CNS & Marna K. Flaherty-Robb, RN, MSN. http://ojin.nursingworld.org/MainMenuCategories/ANAMarketplace/ANAPeriodicals/OJIN/TableofContents/Volume82003/No2May2003/OlderCitizensHealthIssues.html

14. *Healthcare: Millions of Jobs Now and in the Future.* Author: Elka Torpey.
https://www.bls.gov/careeroutlook/2014/spring/art03.pdf

15. *Patient partnership in quality improvement of healthcare services: Patients' inputs and challenges faced.* Authors: Marie-Pascale Pomey, Hassiba Hihat, May Khalifa, Paule Lebel, André Néron. https://pxjournal.org/cgi/viewcontent.cgi?referer=https://www.bing.com/&httpsredir=1&article=1064&context=journal

The following survey is one that local leaders may consider using to survey the health status of their local communities.

Example Community Health Survey

Please take a minute to complete the survey below. The purpose of this survey is to get your opinions about community health problems in (name of jurisdiction). The (name of jurisdiction) Community Health Committee will use the results of this survey and other information to identify the most pressing problems which can be addressed through community action. If you have previously completed a survey, please ignore this. Remember... your opinion is important! Thank you and if you have any questions, please contact us (see contact information on back).

1. In the following list, what do you think are **the three most important factors for a "Healthy Community?"** (Those factors which most improve the quality of life in a community.)

Check only three:

___ Good place to raise children
___ Low crime / safe neighborhoods
___ Low level of child abuse
___ Good schools
___ Access to health care (e.g., family doctor)
___ Parks and recreation
___ Clean environment
___ Affordable housing
___ Arts and cultural events
___ Excellent race relations
___ Good jobs and healthy economy
___ Strong family life
___ Healthy behaviors and lifestyles
___ Low adult death and disease rates
___ Low infant deaths
___ Religious or spiritual values
___ Other ______________________

2. In the following list, what do you think are **the three most important "health problems"** in our community? (Those problems which have the greatest impact on overall community health.)

Check only three:

___ Aging problems (e.g., arthritis, hearing/vision loss, etc.)
___ Cancers
___ Child abuse / neglect
___ Dental problems
___ Diabetes
___ Domestic Violence
___ Firearm-related injuries
___ Heart disease and stroke
___ High blood pressure
___ HIV / AIDS
___ Homicide
___ Infant Death
___ Infectious Diseases (e.g., hepatitis, TB, etc.)
___ Mental health problems
___ Motor vehicle crash injuries
___ Rape / sexual assault
___ Respiratory / lung disease
___ Sexually Transmitted Diseases (STDs)
___ Suicide
___ Teenage pregnancy
___ Other ______________________

3. In the following list, what do you think are **the three most important "risky behaviors"** in our community? (Those behaviors which have the greatest impact on overall community health.)

Check only three:

___ Alcohol abuse
___ Being overweight
___ Dropping out of school
___ Drug abuse
___ Lack of exercise
___ Poor eating habits
___ Not getting "shots" to prevent disease
___ Racism
___ Tobacco use
___ Not using birth control
___ Not using seat belts / child safety seats
___ Unsafe sex
___ Other ______________________

4. How would rate our community as a "Healthy Community?"

___ Very unhealthy ___ Unhealthy ___ Somewhat healthy ___ Healthy ___ Very healthy

5. How would rate your own personal health?

___ Very unhealthy ___ Unhealthy ___ Somewhat healthy ___ Healthy ___ Very healthy

6. Approximately how many hours per month do you volunteer your time to community service? (e.g., schools, voluntary organizations, churches, hospitals, etc.)

___ None ___ 1 - 5 hours ___ 6 - 10 hours ___ Over 10 hours

Please answer questions #7-15 so we can see how different types of people feel about local health issues.

7. Zip code where you live: ___________

8. Age:
   ___ 25 or less
   ___ 26 - 39
   ___ 40 - 54
   ___ 55 - 64
   ___ 65 or over

9. Sex: ___ Male ___ Female

10. Ethnic group you most identify with:
   ___ African American / Black
   ___ Asian / Pacific Islander
   ___ Hispanic / Latino
   ___ Native American
   ___ White / Caucasian
   ___ Other ______________

11. Marital Status:
   ___ Married / co-habitating
   ___ Not married / Single

12. Education
   ___ Less than high school
   ___ High school diploma or GED
   ___ College degree or higher
   ___ Other______________

13. Household income
   ___ Less than $20,000
   ___ $20,000 to $29,999
   ___ $30,000 to $49,999
   ___ Over $50,000

14. How do you pay for your health care? (check all that apply)
   ___ Pay cash (no insurance)
   ___ Health insurance (e.g., private insurance, Blue Shield, HMO)
   ___ Medicaid
   ___ Medicare
   ___ Veterans' Administration
   ___ Indian Health Services
   ___ Other ______________

15. Where / how you got this survey: (check one)
   ___ Church
   ___ Community Meeting
   ___ Grocery Store / Shopping Mall
   ___ Mail
   ___ Newspaper
   ___ Newsletter
   ___ Personal Contact
   ___ Workplace
   ___ Other ______________

Please return completed surveys to the address below by (date). If you would like more information about this community project, please contact us at the number below.

contact name
organization name
address
phone / fax

Thank you very much for your response!

2

Source: file:///Users/reneryman/Downloads/Example-Survey-CTSA-Community-Health.pdf

Notes

Notes

Notes

Notes

Notes

Notes

Notes

Made in United States
North Haven, CT
10 November 2026

22095626R00060